The Only Cure for Healthcare

by

Robert Lalouche, MD, MS

Table of Contents

About the Author

Robert Lalouche, MD, MS is a practicing ObGyn physician for 22 years at the UAP Clinic in Indiana. He received his Undergraduate degree in Electrical and Computer Engineering at the University of California, Davis 1986. He completed his Medical Degree at University of California, Los Angeles in 1991 while simultaneously completing a Master's Degree in Computer Science at UCLA. He completed his Residency at Duke University Medical Center in Obstetrics and Gynecology in 1995 and is a Board Certified ObGyn Physician.

Dr. Lalouche was the founder of ObTech, a mobile software company that won best healthcare software award in 2004. Dr. Lalouche is currently founder and CEO of Doc2Dr, LLC, a Smartphone healthcare software company for the Apple iPhone. www.Doc2Dr.com

Dr. Lalouche has served as High Risk Obstetrics Instructor for the Union Hospital Family Practice Residency where he has won six teaching excellence awards. He served as High Risk Obstetrician for the Maternal Health Clinic, the local indigent care clinic, for approximately 20 years.

Acknowledgments

I thank and acknowledge my wife, Kimberly, for the years of support and patience with my writing endeavor, and for being my loving life partner. I thank my three children, Jeanette, Thomas, and Jack, for the endless joy and challenges they bring me. I thank my mother Fran, whose support and extensive language skills were of great assistance to me in writing this book, and who helped shape the very man I am today. I thank my now deceased father, Guy, who along with my mother, taught me all that I know, especially that hard work and perseverance can conquer any mountain. I thank my sister, Michelle, for helping balance my scientific acumen with human emotions and caring. I thank my best friend, Bill Albert, who is an incredible man and friend, and who has the uncanny skill of finding typos not recognized by any spell checker. I thank Scott Racop, my tennis partner and lawyer friend, who showed me that even a lawyer can be honest and kind. I thank my partner Dr. Sides, who's spirited discussions and insightful views are always welcome. I thank all my friends and family for enduring the many endless discussions and tirades regarding the problems with healthcare and for their invaluable input into this book.

Introduction

There is a real solution to the U.S. Healthcare Crisis, but we are nowhere close to it. Under our current path, Healthcare is the Titanic, and we are just rearranging the deck chairs. Unless the core problem is addressed, no other solution will work. Everyone knows the healthcare system is in crisis, but few recognize a crucial fundamental problem. The overall problem is of course that healthcare costs are rapidly increasing out of control without a matching improvement in quality, access, or outcomes. We provide the best healthcare in the world, yet the cost to provide that care is far higher than all other countries with similar results. To appreciate the real solution, you must first understand the fundamental problem. Let's explore both the obvious and, more importantly, the hidden true problem.

Our country must reduce the cost of care by becoming more efficient - obviously. Many are betting on Electronic Medical Records (EMR/EHR) to improve the efficiency of healthcare, and they can. But, they alone will not solve the core problem of our crisis, and in fact in many ways they are contributors to the problem. Why does it cost so much to produce the results we get? Efficient medical records and exchange of information is crucial, but even the perfect EMR won't solve the real issue. As surprising as it sounds coming from the founder of two medical software companies, we cannot look to EMR's as the core solution, but rather as a secondary, though still important, component of the overall solution.

Everyone deserves a basic level of medical care. If you are in a car wreck, you deserve an ambulance ride to the hospital. If you have cancer, you deserve treatment. If an infection, antibiotics, if high blood pressure, then medications to lower it, if pain, then pain medicine. Happily, whether insured or not, U.S. Healthcare has been providing that to everyone for at least as long as I've been practicing, 25 years, and that's something we can all be proud of. However, we cannot possibly provide unlimited care, medicines, surgeries, diagnostic tests, and interventions without regard to cost, without regard to other equally important needs. We shouldn't perform five tests when one will serve the same purpose, and yet, we do just that. Everyone doesn't deserve a Rolls Royce in their garage and unlimited access to any product their heart desires. So too must there be some limits on the basic healthcare requirements for all individuals. Thankfully, with modest limits and a vast reduction in unnecessary tests and procedures, we can still provide exceptional and efficient healthcare. Interestingly, the excessive unnecessary tests are not the real problem, but rather a side effect of the real problem.

We have tried to limit costs by putting controls in the hands of insurance companies, HMO's, and the government. In some ways, they have had some success, but overall their set of road blocks and hurdles have created more inefficiency, increased costs, and widespread discontent amongst both healthcare providers and patients. This discontent is largely due to the incredible unnecessary waste of everyone's time. They now have a stranglehold on both patients and physicians resulting in escalating premiums for patients and plummeting reimbursement for physicians. Of course, insurance companies are producing revenue for themselves and their shareholders, as any public company is supposed to. I am not suggesting that the insurance companies are the core problem, nor that government healthcare is the solution. Insurance companies are simply passing on the rising costs to the public. Furthermore, their very structure in our system is hampering the usual capitalistic competitive forces that are the cornerstone of successful businesses in the United States. Repairing this competitive imbalance is a key secondary component of the overall solution, just like EMR's, but not the fundamental solution.

Currently in the U.S. we spend far too much to diagnose and treat patient's problems. We spend far too much money on ordering unnecessary and expensive tests with little or no value. We spend far too much time, money, and effort on paperwork to support this excess use of tests and equipment. Paperwork that serves no medical value. We also don't have an effective brake to stop the flood of spending when we know it will be of little additional value. We involve multiple physicians when one or two would do. Our out of control healthcare is the equivalent of the world's most excessive airport transport service. It's like taking a Rolls Royce to the airport with a spare driver, a police escort, 2 back seat drivers, an unlimited supply of food and cocktails, and two separate news crews to record the whole event just in case. It is obvious that we don't need nor deserve such an excessive lavish level of transportation, yet we don't realize that this is exactly what is happening with our healthcare.

The Hidden True Problem

So, why do we spend so much? In two words: defensive medicine. Or, litigation risk. Even without the huge costs of malpractice insurance, its defensive medicine. Simple malpractice reform is not the core solution. To cure healthcare, we need Radical Malpractice Transformation. Let's see how defensive medicine is the fundamental problem, the hidden underappreciated issue, and how Malpractice Transformation is the core solution to the Healthcare crisis.

Some examples should help illustrate how defensive medicine causes extreme overspending.

Example 1: As an ObGyn physician, I get a hospital consult like this at least twice a month. A 23-year-old woman was admitted through the ER with abdominal pain. Her extensive lab results were normal. Her CT scan was normal other than some free fluid in her pelvis, and her ultrasound was normal aside from a small irregular cyst in her ovary. The consulting surgeon doesn't feel she has appendicitis, and the family physician or hospitalist is asking for my consultation. The patient is on expensive IV antibiotics despite a normal temperature, white blood cell count, and infection screen. By the time I'm consulted, she has had 24 to 48 hours' worth of unnecessary tests and exams. I diagnose her with Mittelsmerch (pain of ovulation) and send her home with appropriate follow up plans.

So, how much did this example cost? Well, there were over five physicians – an ER physician, a hospitalist or family physician, a surgeon, an ObGyn, and let's not forget, a radiologist. In fact, there were likely two radiologists. The first who read the CT scan and recommended the ultrasound. Why did they recommend an Ultrasound? CYA Medicine (Cover Your Ass). The second who read the ultrasound, and who will often suggest an MRI for further clarification. (More CYA - if you think I'm joking, just read any radiology report and you'll see I'm not). There were facility fees for the 1-2nights in the hospital. There were IV fluids, IV antibiotics, lab tests including at least a complete blood count, complete metabolic panel, amylase, lipase, pregnancy test (to help decide if there is infection, appendicitis, pregnancy, or other issues). In fact, there might also have been a cardiologist who read the EKG that was ordered because the patient got nervous in the ER, her heart was racing, and she mentioned the dreaded two words "Chest Pain", guaranteed to get you at least an EKG and cardiac labs. Why antibiotics? Well, in case there was an infection that takes some time to clarify. This is not recommended, but often happens as further CYA practices. Furthermore, it won't always get stopped because few want to take responsibility to undue someone else's CYA path. Please note, I don't advocate this, it is just what happens. I will stop it, as will many other more diligent physicians. However, I will have to spend far more time reviewing the entire case to be sure it is the correct decision, rather than taking far less time to leave it as it is. That quicker approach also leaves the responsibility with the originating physician. Virtually no one gets sued for too many treatments, and they surely don't get sued for doing too much. Also, with never ending pressures to get more things done in less time with fewer people, its often just the simple (more expensive) shortcut that is taken. Back to our listing of costs. There are at least 4 nurses – triage nurses, ER nurses, in-hospital nurses. A whole slew of nurses, who provide excellent direct care and comfort for the patient, but who must unfortunately spend far more hours creating at least 5lbs worth of paperwork, consent forms, warning forms, instructional forms, precautionary forms, screening forms to prevent deep vein thrombosis (blood clots in the legs), forms to confirm that in fact the patient was cautioned about the risk of blood transfusion, forms duplicating the same history, forms ensuring that the patient's pain was independently addressed. Forms, FORMS, FORMS! Then there are transcriptionists who must transcribe the dictations of all the involved physicians – history & physical, consults, reports, and final discharge summary. Then there is the utilization review staff, who peruse the chart to help ensure the patient can't be managed out of the hospital. Then there is the compliance review to make sure the patient isn't on inappropriate medicines. Then there is the pharmacist to dispense the medicine. Of course, there are the transporters who handle to and from radiology. Finally, there is the whole team of people who must ensure the paperwork is correctly put together and submitted to the insurance companies for reimbursement. Then there is the team who must go through the chart and find all the missing dates, times and signatures making sure the record is ready for the potential future lawsuit if things are not appropriately signed, dated, and timed. Are you beginning to see the analogy of the Rolls Royce transport with the huge entourage?

How much does all this cost? I venture it ranges from $5,000 to north of $30,000, and easily averages over $10,000 each time. How much should it cost? About $250. Let's see how. First, let's understand what is really happening with the patient.

After spending time seeing the patient, I know the diagnosis thanks largely to skills I first learned from retired Dean Sherman Mellinkoff at UCLA School of Medicine. In his retirement, he took fledgling young medical students around to teach them how important a simple history and physical exam was to medical management. We students were tasked to find him the most difficult, undiagnosed problems in the hospital. With compassion and a laser like acumen, he would often make the diagnosis simply based on his extraordinary skills as a history taker. I was amazed. No tests, no technology, just vast years of experience, knowledge, and the ability to extract a pertinent history of events leading to the present problem. His process was no less amazing than the deductive reasoning of Sherlock Holmes. Fast forward to our young patient and my 25 years of experience. Amongst my many questions, I ask her about birth control pills. Specifically, did she stop? Very often, she will affirm that she recently stopped. Congratulations, we have the diagnosis – Mittelsmerch – pain of ovulation. A very natural and normal physiologic process that happens every month, that can sometimes be very painful, and is often surprising and more painful to women who recently stop taking the birth control pill. (In fact, that's how the birth control pill prevents pregnancy – by stopping ovulation). The process of ovulation involves a growing ovarian cyst (the gradually worsening abdominal ache), that eventually pops (the acute pain that sends the frightened patient to the ER), then regresses leaving behind an irregular cyst and some fluid (seen on the CT Scan and the ultrasound).

Now let's review the same case without defensive medicine, if physicians were free of the worry of being sued, and could practice safe, efficient healthcare.

Example 1 under new system: The same young woman presents to the ER with abdominal pain. Instead of seeing the patient for 30 seconds before ordering labs, scans, and consults, the ER physician performs a thorough history – it would take 5 to 10 precious minutes more. He asks the young woman about her menstrual history and birth control, and quickly discovers she stopped her birth control pills a month ago. His exam finds only mild to moderate tenderness on her left side on pelvic exam, and no signs of infection. Her vital signs are good. He checks an 89¢ urine pregnancy test (not pregnant), screens for STD's, and refers her to follow up with her gynecologist with detailed verbal and written instructions to address possible events before her follow up. He explains that Mittelsmerch – the pain of ovulation - is the most likely diagnosis. She leaves comfortable with a limited prescription for pain medication.

So, how much did it cost this time? The entire encounter probably cost around $250. The majority of the time the ER physician's diagnosis will be correct, and the patient will have been completely cared for at a cost 40 times less. Let that sink in. Forty times less, at minimum.

You may argue that a good ER physician would have done the same efficient encounter under our current system. I would tell you that once any physician has gained enough knowledge and experience to be this good, he also has experienced the sting of being named in a lawsuit. He will know that 99% of the time, this approach will be appropriate. This is by far the most likely cause of her problem; however, the diagnosis is not going to be correct 100% of the time. Rare alternatives are unlikely, but do occur. So, on rare occasion, this patient will have an unusual ovarian tumor, or an atypical appendicitis. In fact, there are at least 20 other less likely possibilities in the differential diagnosis. The current medico-legal requirement forces the physician to excessively pursue these unlikely and extremely rare cases at huge, unaffordable cost overruns. These extra tests are not done anywhere else in the world - you know, in those countries that render equal care for far less.

So, you may argue that the more expensive path prevents that rare missed case. In fact, it doesn't. There is no way to be correct in 100% of cases even if you do every test in existence. However, if you do every test in existence, it will be harder to find you guilty of wrong doing since you did everything available! Here is the root of the problem! To avoid lawsuits and career ruin, not to mention personal shame, physicians are forced to do everything possible to reduce the chance of inappropriate prosecution.

Now, let's follow through the above two examples with the patient having a far less likely underlying diagnosis. Let's say we know ahead of time that the patient has an atypical appendicitis. One with pain on the left instead of the right (it happens). One initially with normal blood tests and no fever. Under the current system, it may get picked up by the CT-scan (but not always). Or, after a day or two in the hospital, the patient will get a fever, her condition will worsen, and under good clinical observation she will get taken to the OR for surgery.

Under the new system I propose, her condition will worsen at home, and then she will return to the ER or her doctor as per the instructions. Her clinical picture will look different, and she will still get the surgery at the same time and have an equally good outcome. However, someone will point fingers and say the original ER doctor made a mistake and should be sued. Perhaps for pain and suffering, or missed work, or delayed diagnosis. The lawsuit may not be successful, because the outcome was good in the end. However, the costs of the lawsuit will still be incurred by the sued physician – not to mention the anxiety and stress of being sued for doing a good job. He or she will be more defensive the next time.

Let's take it further. What about the patient who ignores the instructions and decides to get high on marijuana while at home? Getting high and being surrounded by friends who are high delays her time to surgery. Her appendix ruptures and she dies suddenly before getting back to the hospital. How likely is this? Actually, not very. The astute physician would have assessed her social situation, her risk for noncompliance, and will have adjusted his management accordingly. However, someone will fall through the cracks – IN EVERY SYSTEM, PAST, PRESENT, AND FUTURE – someone will fall through the cracks. The devastated family will fall for a lawyer's commercial offering a large sum of money at no expense and decide to sue. The lawsuit will be for a poor outcome, regardless of whether there was wrong doing. The issue of ignored instructions or illegal drug use will not prevent the lawsuit, though will likely influence the ultimate verdict. The lawyer would claim, if the ER doctor had simply done a CT scan, the patient would have been saved! That is why every doctor must spend the $10,000, even though it doesn't prevent every unnecessary death. We should try for perfection, but having a system that punishes when we don't achieve perfection is harmful and costly. There comes a point where the added effort and cost to completely eliminate all problems is counterproductive. Seeking perfection and achieving it are separate things. Perhaps we should all wear helmets, knee pads, and bullet proof vests all the time? That would reduce injury. Perhaps we should each get a full body MRI every day? That would surely reduce the number of missed illnesses. Who cares that there isn't enough money in the world to pay for this – we can always print more money!

Are you still a skeptic? Perhaps you consider this an unusual fabricated circumstance. Let's delve into other examples with different ways of expressing the same underlying fundamental problem. That fundamental problem being our legal structure that penalizes physicians, even the best of the best physicians, and forces them to practice ridiculously expensive defensive medicine. (By the way, again, this is why we are so much more expensive than other countries that can render similar care cheaper – no country has so many lawyers, and such an out of control legal system – no other country is so lawsuit happy with the deck stacked so high against healthcare providers).

But before we review another example, let's examine another expensive hidden issue. Now we have "Quality Measures", to ensure good performance. One measure is to be sure Emergency Rooms provide quick and efficient care, leaving no one waiting for hours. With cost cutting measures, reduced staff (both physicians and nurses), shortcuts must be taken to meet these "Quality Measures". So, instead of taking a good history, spending time understanding the patient and the problem, the patient is quickly triaged. That is, rerouted to some other doctor or test. If you get your patient out of the ER, in radiology for a CT scan, you've handled the patient and the "quality clock" has stopped ticking. In fact, things have gotten so bad that CT scans are the new abdominal or pelvic exam! That's a VERY costly exam! I have encountered countless patients who have had many CT scans in their teens, yet no physical exam by a physician. These extensive regulatory measures, however well intentioned, take far too much time as currently implemented. More on this issue later, but let's get back to another clinical example. After all, the affordable care act is over 2000 pages, and I'm trying to solve everything in just 50 pages!

The Hidden True Problem: Example 2

Example 2: I am an Obstetrics instructor of Family Practice Residents and the following example is absolutely and unfortunately true. A resident presented this patient to me in the Maternal Health Clinic (our local clinic for indigent pregnant women). She was a 16-year-old pregnant patient at 10 weeks who complained of chest pain at her NOB visit (New Obstetrical). This resident was one of the best, so rather than just waiting for me to make decisions, he demonstrated early initiative and decided to begin the process of working up her chest pain. He ordered Troponins (a blood marker indicative of heart muscle damage and an integral part of diagnosing a heart attack) and an EKG. I was quite surprised, as perhaps you are too. How likely is a 16-year-old to have a heart attack? Giving him the benefit of the doubt, I asked him if she had an underlying heart condition, a congenital heart disease, a strong family history of heart attacks at an early age, some major risk factors like cocaine abuse, etc. All were normal – she was an otherwise normal healthy 16-year-old who just happened to neglect contraception. So, I asked the resident "How likely do you think a heart attack is in this patient?" He said, "Not very likely". I told him to be more specific - 10%? 20%? He said, Zero percent. Really. Zero percent chance she would have a heart attack. Perhaps his percentage was reduced by my tone of inquiry. So, I asked why the hell he ordered a test for a diagnosis he felt was essentially impossible. His response reveals how the Healthcare Titanic is still sinking, still heading in the wrong direction. He said, in the ER, he was taught that if you heard the words "Chest Pain", that you must work up the patient for a heart attack – no debate. Our new Physicians are being taught cook book defensive medicine despite internal protests from their own intellect and common sense. Older frustrated physicians who wouldn't dream of such poor care are retiring, while newer physicians are acclimating to this atrocious system. Can you hear the Titanic's alarms blaring? I asked him to go back and ask the patient if she meant her breasts were sore (a normal symptom in early pregnancy). He did, and she blushingly confirmed that's what she meant. We canceled the tests that would have cost hundreds - the tests that are performed thousands of times per day throughout the country for defensive reasons almost as ridiculous as this case. Try it yourself – go to any ER, tell them you got hit in the chest with a Nerf football or a paintball and you have some mild *CHEST PAIN* – see what happens next. On second thought, don't do it, you may end up with a cardiac catheterization just to be sure, and that has a small but real risk of causing you significant harm. There's enough waste as it is anyway, I don't want to add to it! Besides, without that reflex disclaimer you just read I might be sued too – no kidding, automatic defensive medicine is unavoidable! After all, where else but the USA do you get a coffee cup label with a full paragraph warning about spills and burns?

End of Life issues

OK, let's get back to another example, one very personal to me, that shines the defensive medicine light from a different direction. End of life issues are another area where lawsuits dictate care. I recall one of my senior physician instructors once said, "ah, pneumonia, once the merciful best friend of the elderly". I was perplexed and slightly aghast. He then explained that pneumonia was a merciful death for the very ill and elderly, but that now with super antibiotics and other advanced treatments, we were prolonging the agony of those with virtually no quality of life. My own personal experiences in my family are worth mentioning.

My grandfather, a wonderfully positive influence on my life, died a slow and miserable death from colon cancer when I was in college. At 5'11", he wasted away to under 100lbs at the time of his death. I remember him barely alive in a delirium, grasping my arm with unexpected firmness and pleading: "kill me". That's right, those were his shocking words to me. He wanted desperately to be put out of his misery. I felt so frightened and helpless that I had no words. Later, as a physician in training, I was comforted to know that along with curing illness, I would learn how to provide reassuring comfort care for those near death. How then does this relate to lawsuits? The threat of lawsuits and the excessive provision of useless yet extremely expensive medical care is clearly demonstrated by the death, years later, of my father.

My father, who ironically suggested I become a physician because I would be my own boss (which is far from the current state of medicine), had a rare Lymphoma Cancer of the Skin. He lived well for 9 years of battle with his cancer, then declined in his final year. While leaving the hospital for a chemotherapy visit, he fell and hit his head, receiving a large gash. It was unclear whether a stroke or the spread of cancer led to his fall. You can imagine the hospital staff was frantic, worrying about a fall related lawsuit – but that's not my focus. While standing next to my father, he seemed normal, though muted in his responses. The visiting neurologist asked him if he knew who I was, and to my complete shock and surprise, he did not. Many physicians presented themselves to discuss his case – a neurologist, an oncologist, a neurosurgeon, and an internist. None of them knew him, as they were all covering physicians for the weekend. There was a full court press to provide him with the best care, which I appreciated. The care for a stroke vastly differed from that of metastatic cancer. The option of an open brain biopsy was forwarded as a way to distinguish between the two possible causes. Yes, you heard me. Actually opening up his skull and taking a sample of his brain to analyze! Even as a physician, this seemed barbaric to me. The future outlook was grim either way. Knowing this, and out of the greatest love and respect for my father, I urged the physicians to come up with a simpler, more compassionate, and less invasive way of moving forward with his care. They came up with the option of a brief course of high dose steroids. If it was metastatic cancer, it would temporarily tame the cancer in his brain, and perhaps restore some of his intellect. If it was a stroke, it would have no effect. Pleased with this plan, I went to his home for the night to await the results of this diagnostic procedure. The next morning at 6am, we received a call from my father. He was irritated with us for not coming to pick him up and bring him home. I rushed back to the hospital to see him back to normal, talking to me with clear recognition. This was bittersweet joy, as I had to explain to him that the cancer had spread to his brain, and that this brief return to normal consciousness was very temporary. We shared some tender feelings, then he boldly told me something very crucial. He told me he now knew what the light was that everyone sees before they die. He pointed to the TV at the end of the bed, which was off, and demonstrated that when he turned off the room lights the TV had a faint but clear glow. We both laughed so hard for so long I couldn't tell you if my tears were from joy or sadness. After that, he asked to be taken home – no more tests, no more treatment. I am so happy to say that this time, as compared to my grandfather, I was directly involved in his comfort care during the last few remaining days of his life. So, where is the waste here? Well, there were many offers of MRIs, CT scans, open biopsies, further interventions that easily would have cost $20,000 to $50,000 and more. It was my medical knowledge that allowed me to temper his physicians' natural defensive medical posture. A path, I must say, the physicians greatly appreciated as well.

Let me be more specific, but brief. End of life issues are difficult to address and full of emotions. Many of my readers I'm sure know that a high percentage of all healthcare costs occur within months of one's death. There are caring and compassionate paths open to us all. But, these paths are largely shackled by the threat of lawsuits and not doing "all that is possible". Even when "all that is possible" challenges the Hippocratic Oath of "Above all, do no harm". My purpose here is not to provide all the solutions for end of life issues, but merely to reiterate the enormous additional financial burden our current medic-legal climate causes during this difficult but inevitable part of life.

Lawsuits don't Improve Medical Care

One very crucial point I need to make is that lawsuits, or the threat of lawsuits, don't in anyway make any physician practice better medicine. Let me illustrate. If you're a healthy adult, you're pretty confident in your ability to walk. In fact, I'd say you are an expert. You have years of experience, and you do it well. Every person who walks, however, on rare occasion, stumbles. Perhaps there's a missed curb, or a tree root, or a rock. Or perhaps there's no clear explanation – a stumble just happens. You've stumbled, I've stumbled. There is no human alive who hasn't. Period. If you do stumble, you certainly don't plan it. You're briefly embarrassed, and you move on. If you fall, you pick yourself up. If you get a scrape, you clean it up. No punishment is necessary. The stumble shame is sufficient punishment to deter future stumbles. If I were to suggest to you that we could reduce the number of stumbles and falls if we penalized you with a stiff fine –say 100 times your yearly income - then you would laugh and realize it's ridiculous and wouldn't help. It might make everyone walk slower, more nervously, and perhaps with more caution, but in the end, it would have little or no effect on the number of stumbles and falls. It would make walking a far less efficient means of transportation. In fact, you would likely increase the number of falls by making everyone nervous, tense, and self-conscious. You see where I'm going with this. Huge lawsuits for less than perfect medical outcomes do not improve care in the least. They do not incentivize doctors to do better. They only slow us down and VASTLY increase the cost of healthcare. In fact, in the US, it is my assertion that this is THE reason why your care is so expensive compared to any other country with modern medicine. No other country has such a litigious environment.

One further point regarding the threat of a lawsuit and how it effects a physician's practice patterns. Many who hear my argument suggest that a compromise would be better. That if we just adopted a system of smaller awards, things would work. Or, they point out the great system in Indiana, where I practice, that has a review panel. Lawsuits first go to a panel of peers to evaluate, then the panel renders an opinion. If they render for the physician, it usually ends there. If they render for the patient, it usually gets settled. There is also a compensation fund to tap into. While that reduces huge rewards, it doesn't solve the problem – here's why. Physicians have worked extremely hard all their lives to get to where they are. They are by necessity the top of their class, the hardest workers, the most prolific producers. More important than intelligence is the sheer drive for hard work to achieve the status of physician. Money motivates everyone, including physicians, but excellence and doing great things for people and society are even more important motivators. Every physician wants to be the best.   Suing a physician when they are doing their best for unexpected and arguably unavoidable outcomes is demoralizing. It's not business – its personal. Years ago, medical successes were far fewer, and poor outcomes or death were the unhappy but accepted norm of nature. However, in the last 50 years, our own success in medicine has perhaps become our curse. Most everyone now expects perfection and only great outcomes. If a problem arises, if a bad outcome occurs, then there should be blame, punishment, and shame. That is what our litigious society says. But it is an illusion, and a harmful one. The threat of getting sued NEVER makes me a better doctor, it never makes me practice better medicine, it never motivates me to be more caring and conscientious – nor does it do that for any other doctor I have ever met. As a community of physicians, we all know it. It is our pride that forces us to hide it. We hope to avoid the whole ugly situation by just being perfect, though we know we can't. Many succumb to wasteful defensive practice patterns of "do everything" to avoid lawsuits. Those of us who don't, still observe and work with those wasteful patterns on a daily basis. Few physicians start this way. We all start out idealistic and proud. We all practice as we are taught. We are taught that if we are friendly, caring, attentive, and hardworking, we will not get in a lawsuit. Then reality hits, and we slowly evolve into defensive practices, or at least tolerate the entire system of defensiveness that we know is a ridiculous waste of time and money. I have been named in many lawsuits, but none successful. Every lawsuit I have been named in is when I have done some of my best medicine. Bad things, however, still happen. Nature is the real boss – we just tame her a bit. I love this quote from the movie World War Z – "Mother Nature is a serial killer. No one's better. Or more creative." We all strive for perfect healthcare, but just as sure as we walk and sometimes stumble, we will always have only near perfect outcomes.

I slipped in an enigma you may not have even noticed. How is it possible that some of my best work has resulted in lawsuits? Let me explain by example. My wife was in labor years ago, resting comfortably with her epidural at 3am. I was the attentive husband and father to be, not the physician caring for my wife. I left our labor room to stretch my legs and noticed an emergency. A laboring woman walked in near delivery with a breech baby (feet first). This situation most often warrants an emergency cesarean section. While the physician on call, my wife's physician, was 20-30minutes away, I was right there and could resolve the emergency in minutes. So, the resident set up for a C-section, while I conferred with my wife. With her approval, I assumed responsibility for the emergency, as any good Samaritan would. When I went back out of our labor room to begin the C-section, there was a new unnatural quiet to labor and delivery and no one to be found. I scanned the monitors and noticed a new arrival with a worrisome fetal heart rate in the 70's (much too low for a baby, and if persistent, a sign of imminent death). Two new emergencies virtually at the same time! I stepped in the new room to find the resident, and all eyes were on me to act. I was the most capable to take charge and immediately took action – some of my finest work as a physician. We summoned the on-call physician, while adjusting our cesarean plans to this new more emergent patient. I then examined the patient and assessed that using a vacuum then forceps could potentially expedite the delivery instead of a cesarean. This risky maneuver may succeed in a woman who's had a prior delivery. I was able to deliver the baby that way – it worked! Two minutes from when I met this patient, and under 10minutes from when she walked in the door, I had successfully delivered the baby. The on-call physician came in and delivered the other baby by C-section. A success all around...almost.

The baby I delivered never had a heart rate above 70, and was pronounced dead within the hour. It was already too late before we got started. So, there's the lawsuit – a neonatal death. A horrible tragedy. But no, there was no lawsuit. You see, the couple who just met me, who saw me do my best, despite their sorrow, thanked me. They knew I had done something heroic. They knew I wasn't their doctor and yet still came to their rescue. They knew I wasn't even on call or on duty. They knew no one else could have moved any faster. They thanked me and even decided to come to me as their doctor for their future pregnancy. So, where is the lawsuit? Well, remember Nature and her creativity? The couple's next child turned out to have a lethal birth defect. One that is uniformly fatal, but not until delivery. The couple delivered 9 months later at a tertiary center, and of course, their second baby subsequently died. I assume the emotional burden of two horrible tragedies and significant expenses, motivated them to sue. They decided to sue their original doctor for the first fetal demise. With lawyers, everyone gets pulled in. So, here is my lawsuit, from the couple who thanked me for doing my best. After all, it's only business, only money. But from then on, I had to list the pending lawsuit. I had legal expenses. I had the enormous psychological burden of knowing that everyone, under the right circumstances, will turn to a lawyer and sue. To pay their bills. To blame someone. To lash out in understandable pain and sorrow. The lawsuit was not successful, but the damage was done. I now know, as all physicians eventually find out, that no matter how good you are, the specter of a lawsuit and the huge financial and emotional toll it takes, is always there. If this specter were eliminated, if physicians could be free to practice sound medicine without persecution for being mere mortals, not gods, then even higher quality healthcare could be had for far less. We could provide reasonably priced exceptional medicine for everyone.

Physicians Hate Healthcare Software

Most Healthcare Providers absolutely hate EMRs (Electronic Medical Records), EHRs (Electronic Health Records), CPOE (Computer Physician Order Entry), and virtually all software used for healthcare. Are all providers inept when it comes to software? Absolutely not. The real problem is that software is designed for insurance companies, billing companies, lawyers, the government, and "Big Data" collectors, not to enhance the doctor patient relationship or to make physicians more efficient. Virtually all medical software wastes providers' time rather than saves it. Not only that, with each iteration, and more rules and regulation, the inefficiency and waste is growing, not shrinking. Speaking for every physician I know, this must stop!

This disdain might seem odd coming from a computer scientist/physician – after all, I'm definitely a computer geek. However, as a physician, I want computers and software to help me, not hinder me. I know how it should be, I know how it can be, and it is nowhere close. That makes me even more disdainful for the egregious, unnecessary interruption of the Doctor Patient relationship. The current implementation of medical software is so far from being of help that it is an embarrassment and a further step toward the total collapse of the healthcare system.

You see, EMR's and CPOE are geared toward documenting things in perfect detail for the inevitable lawsuit when things don't go perfectly. Everything clearly shown, dated, timed, and repeatedly signed by the physician is the perfect prosecutors tool. That's right, the current configuration of all the computer systems are mostly tailored for lawyers, insurance companies, and the government to be able to accuse, sue, or bill, or prove false billing. Not, I repeat, not, to provide good healthcare for patients.

Before EMRs and CPOE, there were preprinted order protocols and paper charts. If I had an uncomplicated patient for surgery, I would sign the routine post op orders in 3 seconds. Now, with CPOE, that takes 5-10 minutes – soon, with a new software "upgrade", it will take longer. For rounding, I would review the chart for progress, labs, vitals, then go see the patient. Afterwards, I would document in the chart the patient's routine progress. This whole process for a routine patient would typically take 5 to 15 minutes, with the majority of the time spent face to face with the patient. Now, with EMRs and CPOE, you would think it would be even simpler, more efficient, and faster. You would be dead wrong. It takes double or even triple the time. There are so many hurdles, regulations, and additional unnecessary steps in software geared for those regulators, billers, and lawyers, that it takes much more time. So many things that ancillary staff used to take care of are now the job of physicians to handle. Why are we forced to be billers, coders, cashiers and data entry personnel? In the past, billing fraud from a few bad apples created the legal requirement for physicians to enter, sign, and date every single order. The reasons are a poor solution to prevent fraud, rather than a smart efficient solution to help patients. I could write an entire book on this topic alone. Suffice it to say, the lawsuit-government-insurance-guided direction is the wrong direction. We need an immediate 180-degree U-turn to save our sinking healthcare ship. Later, we'll see how we can resolve this software problem with a major refocus of medical software toward enhancing the care of patients and the efficiency of physicians.

The Cure

Complaining about the problem and even identifying its root cause is not enough to cure it. Here's a high-level overview of the path to the cure. There are likely additional helpful components to a real cure, however, without fundamentally changing our approach to lawsuits in medicine, I guarantee no other solution will work.

1. **Reinstate the Good Samaritan law for hospitals and healthcare workers, with transparency and structured assessment for improvement.**
2. **Agree on a fair but affordable basic level of healthcare that everyone is entitled to and that is paid for by everyone for everyone in taxes. (sales tax, income tax, sin tax, etc.). Most importantly, we must have a budget for it and the numbers must balance.**
3. **Private Insurance is for extra services above and beyond the basic.**
4. **Apply the same Good Samaritan law to Pharmaceutical and Medical device companies with transparency in personal responsibility.**
5. **Allow free market competitive forces to work their magic.**
6. **Eliminate the middle men from healthcare – insurance companies and the government are no longer in the middle. Doctors with patients make care decisions.**
7. **Provide paths for healthier living and consequences for not.**
8. **No one gets a free ride. No one. Everyone gets to share in the pride of contributing.**
9. **Refocus Software for Physicians and Patients, Not Insurers and the Government**

Solution: Reinstate the Good Samaritan law

U.S. Healthcare costs as a percentage of GDP have risen from under 5% for our entire history until the early '60s when the Good Samaritan law was removed as umbrella protection for Hospitals and when Medicare and Medicaid were established. Since that time, this percentage has steadily grown now to almost 20%

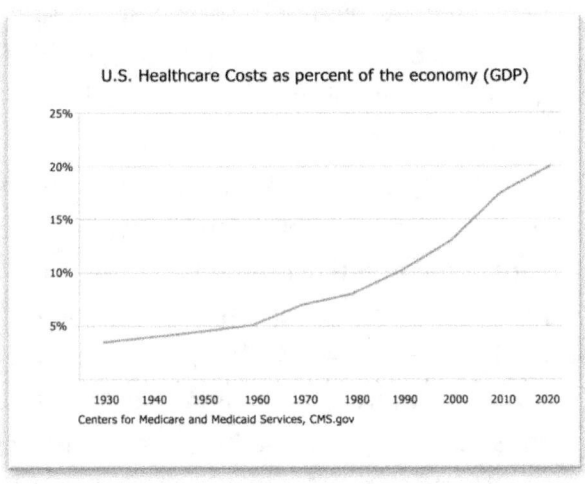

Reducing and especially eliminating out of pocket expenses has led to over utilization and increased costs, but lawsuits are also the indirect factor too often underestimated. Removing lawsuits for physicians and hospitals will tame the beast.

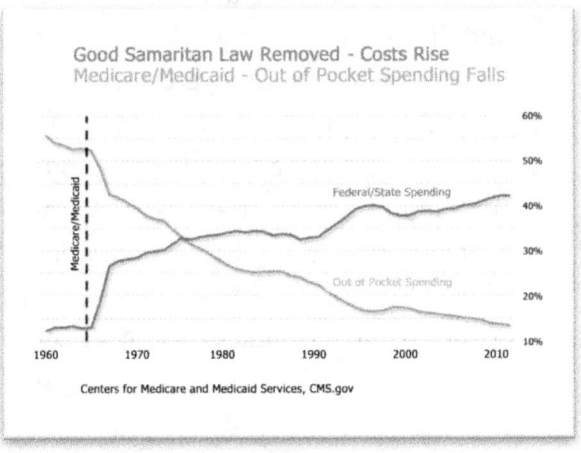

It will allow the practice of evidence based medicine, rather than "everything-based" medicine.

There will necessarily be some training, some retooling, and much transitional guidance. Those details will be left for another publication, for now I must address the obvious concern about individual patient welfare. The answer to that is transparency. Publication of patient anonymous statistics regarding outcomes and complications will serve as the check and balance. For patients with inadvertent poor outcomes, care will be provided to remedy the situation. There will be no pot of gold for lawyers or patients, since the lawsuit does not incentivize any physician or hospital to give better care. There will be panels to assess any medical error or poor outcome. There will be monitoring, evaluation, and non-judgmental remediation. If a physician is a repeat offender of sub-par care and corrective intervention fails, he or she will lose that privilege. For sub-par performance on an individual level for healthcare workers, nurses, staff, physicians, all the way up to hospitals, there will be instruction and sharing of success from those who perform the best. The spirit of medical school and residency is one of training, sharing, and betterment for all. Why should that cease upon entry into the real world? You wouldn't think it's the case, and yet egos, competition, and excessive time consuming paperwork largely prevent that cooperative learning and continuous improvement amongst physicians. With integrated continuous cooperation and sharing of ideas, far better results for all can result. By focusing on the positive and eliminating the unproductive punitive environment of lawsuits, we can raise the quality of care while drastically reducing healthcare costs.

Solution: Basic Healthcare for All

Let me point out something you may not realize if you believe the media's distorted portrayals of Healthcare in the United States. Everyone gets the essential care they deserve – insurance or not. Anyone can walk in to any hospital and get emergency care. As a physician, I provide hundreds of thousands of dollars in medical care to patients every year that never gets reimbursed. I believe everyone will agree that there is a basic level of care that we are all entitled to. That basic level needs to be defined, and it needs to be affordable. If you get into a car wreck and break your arm, well then you deserve a cast. If you get cancer, you deserve basic cancer treatment. Do you deserve a single room with free cookies like a grand hotel? No. (cookies are the newest bonus at hospitals to coax good evaluations and patient satisfaction surveys – what an incredibly poor application of hotel management principals). Do you deserve an expensive experimental treatment with virtually no chance of success? No. Recently, I heard of a new drug that costs $70,000 and has been shown to extend a stage 4 cancer patient's life for six months – is everyone entitled to that – no. That's what private insurance is for. How about lung cancer treatment if you are a smoker? Well, here is an opportunity. Let's heavily tax cigarettes to pay for that. Or set some limits here. Such measures would actually benefit smokers financially if they quit.

How about epidurals? Should that be covered for everyone? Epidurals are very effective but also expensive so it is with great difficulty that I suggest it may be optional. These are some of the tough decisions we must face. However, if I'm to choose between cancer care for everyone, and cheaper

IV pain medicines over epidurals, so be it. I'm certain that every physician in every specialty can rank medical treatments and interventions based on how essential their universal availability is. Based on such rankings, a budget can be applied, and that is what we get. We must stop living beyond our means as a nation, or we will go bankrupt.

Solution: Private Insurance is for Extras

Do you want a private room? Do you want that extra MRI just in case? Do you want the new branded drug rather than a generic? That's what private insurance is for. Do you want infertility care, or medicines for erectile dysfunction? That's for private insurance. Do you want a heart transplant at 75? An experimental treatment for lung cancer after all other proven methods have failed? That's for private insurance. Do you want a hospitality cookie or a gourmet meal at the hospital? That's for your pocket book or private insurance. How about elective cosmetic surgery? You get the message. There is much medical care that can be excluded from our base allotment that allows everyone to get the best healthcare in the world, without bankrupting our country. We're way overboard now by ordering almost everything for everyone simply to avoid lawsuits. Many more patients can be accommodated with semiprivate rooms, but are not as a result of HIPAA privacy issues. It is nice to have a private room with a private bathroom, but is everyone entitled to it? We have to prioritize and decide where to devote our funds. Excessive attention to HIPAA is costing our country a lot, and yet not really delivering perfect privacy. Avoidance of HIPAA violations lawsuits cost far more than just using common courtesy. Just recently I overheard a nursing meeting that focused on extraordinary measures to avoid rare human errors where some paper work went to the wrong place, causing large lawsuits. This meeting occurred next to a newly remodeled recovery room area which had sound proof glass enclosures rather than curtains, for HIPAA concerns. We all value privacy, but really to have one hundred percent privacy for everyone, each hospital could only serve one patient at a time! After all, if you see another patient in the hall, that reveals that they are receiving medical care. Ridiculous you say, well, that's how ridiculous some of our expensive efforts are in the name of privacy. No other country goes to such extremes – we as a country have to decide if that's where we should divert our funds. Healthcare for all children, treatment for all cancers, birth control for all, or ultra-privacy for everyone. The excess focus on HIPAA is lawsuit driven. To summarize, we need to agree on what is affordable fair basic coverage for everyone.

Solution: Pharmaceutical Companies

Yes, I know this is quite controversial. Hollywood, the press, and lawyers have done a great job of casting Big Pharma as supervillains out to get a buck at the expense of anyone's life. Sure, perhaps a few bad apples haven't helped. However, the same companies, the people and scientists and engineers and administrators behind the companies, have done incredible things to make our lives better, longer, and safer. They deserve our thanks and respect, not our fear and derision.

So, why do drugs cost so much and take so long to get out? Lawsuits. A high percentage of new drugs and medical products get pulled or recalled due to lawsuit frenzies. Frenzies created by deceitful, greedy lawyers hiding behind empty claims of protecting the public. Many suits are for bad outcomes from known and stated potential side effect. I waste hours every day talking to patients about lawsuit-fanned problems. (Surgical Mesh, Birth Control Pills, Intra Uterine Devices, Antibiotics, Diabetic Medicines – the list is endless, these are just some I must address on a daily basis).

Here is the solution outlined:

- No lawsuits allowed against drugs or drug companies that comply with full transparency of study data, design, complications, side effects, etc. Patients are fully informed, and can then accept the risk with the hope to achieve the benefit. The same holds for Medical Device Companies.
- Instead, there should be criminal proceedings against company members, not just companies, for any falsified information. If any company or employee hides or falsifies

information, then the risks and benefits cannot be fairly represented. A patient who suffers consequences as a result of this lie should get the care to resolve it, while the perpetrator goes to court. There is no need for a pot of gold. The pot of gold only encourages trolling lawyers, raises costs, and encourages defensive medicine.

- No company can be sued for an FDA approved drug for a side effect or complication found and disclosed in the studies. New problems/side effects cannot be sued for either – they will be assessed, then appropriate measures will be taken to ensure safety.

- End ridiculous drug commercials that are forced to emphasize the side effects and risks instead of the benefits. This is confusing and misleading to patients. Patients are more likely to avoid these medicines that would help them due to excessive warnings. However well intentioned, these warnings are doing far more harm than good.

- End lawyer commercials trolling for "patients" and effectively rendering medical advice. Patients are too frightened to use perfectly great products due to these trolling commercials, and hence suffer worse medical outcomes. I have countless numbers of patients who have suffered the horrible consequences of osteoporosis, including disability and death, due to avoiding the use of medications for extremely rare risks of problems with their jaw. A 70-year-old patient who breaks a hip has a 50% chance of death within a year due to complications, but well under 1% risk of serious jaw problems (osteonecrosis of the jaw). Many patients simply avoid care for that irrational fear.

I now have the dubious privilege of participating in a class action deposition against a medical device company regarding an exceptional product. I was merely a witness of fact regarding a patient. The suit targets a great product I have used successfully for many years, and continue to use today. Unfortunately, the better a product is, the more widely it is used, the more likely it will be the target of a trolling lawyer. It's simple math – the popular product will eventually result in that rare side effect. This is the target of class action lawyers. It's the Sutton principal, name after Willie Sutton. When asked why he robbed banks, Willie stated "That's where the money is". For the vast majority of these cases, lawyers pretend to be the savior for the meek and injured. Instead they are motivated by vast fees, indifferent to the incredible boost in price of all medical products. The money has to come from somewhere. Why else would a $2 piece of plastic (IUD) cost $750?

Solution: Free Market Competitive Forces

The long history of economic leadership in the US is evidence enough of the benefits of capitalism and the free market economy. With healthcare being the largest segment of the economy, it still amazes me how many controls, regulations, and barriers there are that interfere with this proven concept. Transparency as proposed throughout this book should help. Allowing insurance coverage to cross state lines will too. As a physician, it is incumbent upon me to practice excellent, cost-conscious medicine. However, with such a complex and "hidden" system, choosing the least expensive amongst equally viable paths for care is extremely difficult. Both patients and healthcare providers have no clear and simple path to be able to understand their costs and make decisions based upon them. Transparency of quality measures should also extend to costs transparency.

Let's simplify for example. If you shop for a plain sweater, and find it costs $500, you won't buy it. If it costs $50, it is probably ok. If it costs $5, and is worth $50, then everyone will buy it and the sweater company goes bankrupt. With healthcare today in the U.S, no one knows the cost or the value – not doctors, nurses, patients, hospital execs, not even insurance companies or pharmaceutical companies. There are hidden contracted rates, across the board discounts. With our sweater example, many people will get charged $5,000, but have a contracted discount to pay a co-pay of only $50. Others have no coverage, work hard, but can't afford $5,000, so go without a sweater and get cold. Others have no money, don't work, and get theirs for free. Those who work but can't afford the sweater wonder why, decide to stop working, so someone else can pay for their free sweater. To summarize, it is very difficult to comparison shop when the price is obfuscated. Furthermore, it is very difficult to comparison shop when quality is not clearly evident. We have a system that conceals excellence in physicians and limits competition based on the quality of service.

By treating physicians as commodities, we prevent real differentiation based on service, and have an extremely poor substitute in the form of quality measures. Internet evaluation sites are seriously flawed, and often devolve into complaint sites. Personality and bed side manner are certainly important, though public evaluations based solely on this measure support poor physicians with great personalities and penalize great physicians with only average personalities. Other objective measures can certainly help. Non-judgmental complication rates for facilities and physicians will help reduce costs by competitive forces as well as help provide acceptance with lawsuit restrictions. When the public sees that complications, though infrequent, are realities of every business, including the business of healthcare, then there will be more acceptance. Show me a physician who has never had any complications, and I'll show you a physician who has no experience. The path to excellence is always tortuous and bumpy.

In a more open and transparent environment, those who achieve such excellence can bring others along their path. Due to the threat of lawsuits and the stigma of imperfection, physicians virtually cease to assist each other along the never-ending learning path. Restructuring our current system away from huge monetary punishments and toward leaders teaching followers will raise the quality for everyone. For example, ask any surgical tech in any operating room in the country and they can immediately tell you which surgeon or surgeons are the "best" for a certain procedure, and which have something to be desired. Is there any built-in mechanism to get the physician with excellence to assist the learner? No, not enough. Time, money, and attention should be diverted in this direction, rather than toward huge lawsuits for imperfect outcomes. I practice in a multi-specialty group and my partners and I strive for such interactions and group self-improvement, but the entire culture of healthcare has room for much improvement in this area.

Solution: Eliminate the Middle Men

Healthcare providers waste far too much time complying with and pandering to insurance company and government hurdles. Hurdles of documentation, billing and coding, consent forms, sign/dating, well intentioned blanket quality guidelines, and more. We need to cut these middle men out of the doctor patient relationship. They need to be on the sidelines. Electronic Medical Records are designed to be the instruments to pander to these requirements, rather than simple effective tools to assist and expedite physician's quality care.

Nurses spend as little as 15% of their time face to face with patients and physicians as little as 25%. At least double that is spent with paperwork, charts, and EMRs. Those numbers can and should be reversed, but they can't be with all the extreme requirements of documentation created in large part for the benefit of lawyers, not patients or healthcare workers. As the CEO of a startup software company, I am striving to create software solutions that save healthcare providers time, not waste it. Large EMR companies need a complete reroute of priorities, but they can't do it now in our current medico legal climate.

Insurance submissions are not for healthcare providers to perform; they are an issue between the patient and the insurance company. The basic level of service covered by the government can be simplified, streamlined, and largely automated if done correctly. Patient's should handle the claims to extra private insurance, or pay doctor's offices for that service. This will provide a good transition for the large employee base devoted to insurance and billing processing.

Let's examine a well-intentioned quality measure and show how it wastes time and money. Under "Obamacare", every patient is supposed to get a summary printout of their visit. In my multispecialty group of about 100 physicians, the ink and paper costs alone of these handouts per year easily amount to about $100,000. Guess what happens to the majority of those handouts? You guessed it, they end up in the trash can of our office – before the patients even leave! What happens if we stop printing them? We lose money from the government for not meeting the quality measures. Now, suppose I have a 90-year-old patient on multiple medications, and today I modify one of those medicines. She's a perfect candidate for a reference handout, and I don't need the government to tell me I should provide it for her. However, as you recall, I'm an Obstetrician. I see a pregnant patient approximately 13 times in 30 weeks, including weekly in the last month. How useful do you think they find a weekly printout showing them they are pregnant and taking prenatal vitamins? Can you say trash can liner? Certainly, large research bodies can give advice on protocols for great healthcare, but ultimately it should be up to the healthcare provider to decide if it applies, and such a high-level binding of reimbursement and quality measures inevitably leads to wasted time and money. The one size fits all approach wastes so much money, as we see in the failings of communism with high level edicts and no low level competitive forces.

Solution: Provide paths for healthier living

We have so many freedoms in the US that make life great that I would never suggest we forbid someone from smoking so long as it doesn't harm others. However, there is no reason I or any other American should pay for the poor health choices of others. So, if someone decides to smoke, we should withhold something sufficient to cover the extra healthcare costs of that choice, which are quite high. Why should we give food stamps or welfare to someone who plans to puff it away in smoke? We should provide smoking cessation help for free (as we largely do now). We should tax cigarettes high enough to pay for their expensive unhealthy consequences. If they can afford cigarettes, they don't need financial assistance. Cigarettes are one of the best ways to keep a poor person poor, and yet we applaud that harmful freedom. Sure, if you want to smoke, it's your right. But others shouldn't have to pay for your unhealthy choice. As a physician, I am regularly asked to write a prescription for inexpensive over-the-counter medicines (like allergy medicines, or stool softeners, or vitamins) to Medicaid patients. They request them because with a prescription, they will be free (paid for by John Q Taxpayer). I politely let them know that they merely need to avoid smoking for a day to easily pay for the medication.

As a physician, my scope of care frequently extends to social, emotional, and financial issues. Many of my most successful methods of encouraging people to quit smoking, usually for patients in their 40's who feel poor and "stuck" financially, is to point out financial realities. I demonstrate how cigarettes are stealing their American dream and keeping them stuck in debt in addition to burning away their health.

I've had three patients quit smoking when I offered them a free trip to Hawaii in a year, paid for with their saved money by quitting smoking.

The United States has a long tradition of encouraging behavior using tax incentives. That's why there are tax breaks for marriage, or starting a new business. I think we should seriously consider taxes to encourage healthier eating as well. I have many patients who receive government aide in the form of cheap, unhealthy foods. Perhaps we should provide discounts on fresh fruits and vegetables and taxes on fast food and sugar loaded drinks. Do I believe we should ban high calorie foods – of course not. I for one love a few unhealthy foods on occasion, and I love that I live in a country where I get such a wide selection and I have the freedom to choose. However, I find it very reasonable to encourage healthier eating and to make healthy eating available to everyone in our country by incentivizing with well-placed sales taxes and discounts.

Solution: No one gets a free ride

Free rides are unfair and costly, and psychologically harmful to the recipient. Everyone likes a "freebie", but imagine if you never had to earn a thing? I submit to you that one of life's greatest joys is enjoying the fruits of your hard work. Everyone has the ability to contribute in some way to the cost of their healthcare, and yes, I do mean everyone. Does that mean we withhold care if someone can't pay – absolutely not – remember, we should and already do receive a basic level of healthcare. However, we should all contribute in some form or another. Payments, volunteer time, community clean up, even a cigarette exchange. That's right, if you smoke, you should have to leave your pack of cigarettes as collateral until you can pay.

A colleague of mine reminded me of how less opulent countries require that any hospitalized patient must provide a "care giver" who cooks all their meals, bathes them, and assists in any other way. Some similar form of support could be implemented here, allowing family and friends to share in the pride of contributing.

Free rides and no barriers to healthcare have enormous costly effects on our system of healthcare. There are many patients who regularly go to emergency rooms for no reason other than they can go to get immediate care and have nothing to pay. There must be some barrier to prevent overuse. Obamacare, with far more insured lower income individuals, hasn't changed the habits of this large core of patients – many will still take an ambulance ride to the ER for a minor health issue.

Right now, with very high deductibles for patients who pay for insurance, we have an unusual paradox. The money for high premiums and huge deductibles is paying for the lower income individuals to get their care for free. However, with no barrier, these individuals are getting far more healthcare, while the high deductible patients are opting to avoid screening procedures, non-life threatening procedures, or routine healthcare. The paradox is those who pay nothing are getting better healthcare than those who pay the most. If no one gets a free ride, if everyone must contribute in some way, this balance can normalize to fair basic healthcare for everyone.

Solution: Refocus Healthcare Software

Software has the potential to save physician's time, rather than waste it. With integrated medical intelligence, it can increase the amount of time physicians spend with patients, rather than interfere with it. Eliminating lawsuits and excessive government and insurance controls will help vastly. My software company is focused on saving physicians time under the current environment. Most current healthcare software is focused on meeting the billing and coding guidelines, regulatory guidelines, and quality measures. This focus creates forests of data that obscure the important medical information. This over documentation reduces quality, rather than improving it.

"Big data" is the exciting new frontier, with deep analysis of massive quantities of medical data. The major barrier now is that physicians are burdened with ever increasing, timing wasting, data entry which raises costs and impedes the doctor patient relationship. New "improved" diagnostic codes have increased fivefold from 13,000 to 68,000. This enhanced diagnostic granularity is needed for better data analysis. However, it has magnified the data entry requirements for physicians, further cutting into patient time. Think of that the next time you see your physician for seconds instead of minutes. There is a way to avoid this, but current medical software doesn't address it well. With the changes I propose, there is a clear path to streamlining this data input. Perhaps an analogy will help illustrate. Big data is like having a Ferrari three hundred years ago. It looks promising, but without the simple infrastructure of paved roads, it will go nowhere fast. Simple software with medical intelligence that automatically collects big data can create the roadway infrastructure needed to allow that big data Ferrari to race to success.

Healthcare software is such a large topic, that I will limit the discussion by saying we need a completely different path toward success. A path as radically different, and simple, as the iPhone was compared to all phones before it. Every physician knows current software impedes rather than helps them. There is nothing that proves this further than the surge in expletives that can be heard with each new increasingly burdensome software "upgrade".

The Elephant in the Room

The elephant in the room is that Radical Malpractice Transformation will likely be fervently opposed by lawyers. With the majority of congressman being lawyers, this is no baby elephant. Furthermore, lawyers do not create lawsuits alone, so our citizens will also hesitate to relinquish any control. I do not suggest we eliminate individual rights and protections. There are alternatives to ensuring those crucial elements remain. Transparency, criminal cases for egregious violations, to name a few. I believe most lawyers are reasonable and logical, and also want great healthcare at a reasonable cost for the public, including themselves. Things can be simplified, even with lawyers. We can make the changes now, or we can wait until the Titanic is on the ocean floor. The choice is ours. Recently, I reviewed the requisite surgical risks with a patient, including the ridiculous, useless details required by law (think any drug commercial) and my patient summed it up quite nicely. She said, the consent should read: "Your surgery is Cesarean section. Shit happens." I doubt we could ever get that simple, but it's worth a try!

Doctors are Human Too

Many of my family and friends suggested that the tone of this book was too angry. It turns out, they were right. (Yes, you are reading the toned-down version). You see, when you dedicate your life to work hard to help others, to save lives, you look forward to thanks and appreciation. The successes are reward enough, but as most physicians will tell you, the thanks, the smile, the hug, the genuine appreciation, is the real reward of being a healthcare provider. The reward of helping others makes those years of endless nights of studying and hard work, the enormous and numerous sacrifices, all worth it. Then you are sued. Sued for a bad outcome, not negligence. Sued for the unavoidable stumble. Sued for the realities of life, at your finest moment. Then, resentment, anger, and many other human emotions come in to play. After all, doctors are human too. Many studies report physician burn out rates ranging from 30% to 60% - an increasing amount overtime. Our current medico-legal climate is a great contributor to this problem, which expands on the increasing costs of medicine. Have you heard of a physician shortage? Ask any physician if they recommend the same career path for their children. That recommendation has been decreasing too.

If a stock broker picks the wrong stock, do we sue them for all they are worth? How about if a movie star forgets their lines? How about a janitor, or a banker, or a lawyer? Of course not. We don't expect perfection. We want it, but when we don't get it, we forgive and move on. How about for a Policeman? Oh, that opens up another can of worms. There's another underappreciated group. Suffice it to say, the higher the stakes, the less forgiving we are. Yet no matter how high the stakes, we are all imperfect humans.

If we can come up with a healthcare system that encourages the strive for perfection, yet constructively handles the bumps along the road, we can boost morale, reduce costs, and achieve new heights of quality care for everyone.

This chapter was finished, until something highly germane happened to me today. A new junior partner called for help during a particularly difficult hysterectomy. With the help of two other gynecologists and a general surgeon, the surgery went very well. As I was walking down the hall feeling pleased with the outcome, it happened. My analogy came to life, and I stumbled. Right there, in the hall, with no twig or rock, I had a very slight stumble. I didn't fall, but it was a humbling reminder. I laughed at myself and smiled. Then, it reminded of a recent lawsuit I was involved with, a suit with a bowel injury. A suit where I performed at my finest. A surgery with a stumble. Followed by a timely correction.

Only human.

Conclusion

It may be controversial to claim that the only cure to healthcare is a fundamental change in our approach to lawsuits in medicine. There are certainly many other improvements with promise that I have not included here, yet none will come close to resolving our crippled system without the changes I suggest. Clearly, we need to be able to set limits on healthcare spending. Eliminating defensive medicine will help significantly in that regard. However, setting healthcare limits will still remain a difficult issue, especially when individual lives are at stake. If we don't face these issues, however, then catastrophic financial consequences are around the corner. These consequences will have far more impact on the health and wellbeing of everyone. Let's stop shuffling the chairs on the Titanic and really fix this problem together. The only cure for healthcare requires radical malpractice transformation, deregulation, and the restoration of competition.